MEMORIES OF A YOUNG PHARMACIST
TALES OF TENDER CARE

BEVERLY CLARK

outskirtspress
DENVER, COLORADO

The opinions expressed in this manuscript are solely the opinions of the author and do not represent the opinions or thoughts of the publisher. The author has represented and warranted full ownership and/or legal right to publish all the materials in this book.

Memories of a Young Pharmacist
Tales of Tender Care
All Rights Reserved.
Copyright © 2015 Beverly Clark
v4.0

Cover Photo © 2015 Beverly Clark. All rights reserved - used with permission.

This book may not be reproduced, transmitted, or stored in whole or in part by any means, including graphic, electronic, or mechanical without the express written consent of the publisher except in the case of brief quotations embodied in critical articles and reviews.

Outskirts Press, Inc.
http://www.outskirtspress.com

ISBN: 978-1-4787-3848-0

Outskirts Press and the "OP" logo are trademarks belonging to Outskirts Press, Inc.

PRINTED IN THE UNITED STATES OF AMERICA

Table of Contents

1: Overzealous Student 1

2: Patient Counseling - Very Patient! 5

3: Burying the Hatchet 8

4: Behind Closed Doors 14

5: The Doctor and The Fly 20

6: The Perfect Gentleman 25

7: His Kingdom for a Car Ride 27

8: The Kiss 30

9: Drugstore Robbery 34

10: Til Death Do Us Part 39

11: Can We Be Honest? - Selling Clinical Services 42

12: The Doctor who refused to grow old 48

1
Overzealous Student

Poor Vicki suffered from that dreadful malady called the "overzealous student syndrome." It was obvious to all who knew her, but no one knew what to do about it. Most conscientious pharmacy students suffered from the same disease for a short period, but mercifully nature and reality slowly and gently brought the student around until a spontaneous cure was realized.

Why this particular girl could not overcome the syndrome puzzled even her college professors. "Surely, she realizes that we're not that serious!" they whispered among-themselves when they watched the small figure stumbling about campus, the slender arms overloaded with Goodman & Gilman, Harrison's Textbook of Medicine, Hansten's Drug Interactions and <u>Applied Therapeutics</u>.

Even Dr. Marley, the most extreme proponent of pure professionalism finally became concerned. Naturally, in the best interests of professionalism he simply could not abandon the party line. Or else the other students, not infected with Vicki's illness, wouldn't even bother to show up for class. Besides, if word got out, he might even lose his job. But there was something appealing about little Vicki, in her malady, that touched old Dr. Marley's heart.

Seeing this female student burdened with pharmacy textbooks and notecards containing the chemical structures of the terpenes brought the professor of pharmacognosy back to the days when his every word had been listened to and revered. That was when his children were still toddlers. He would quote to them from pharmacy journals as they sat upon his knees, looking into his face with innocent, adoring eyes. Now, adults themselves, they found his discussions frankly boring and repetitive.

But in the eyes of this female student, Dr. Marley still saw adoration. Vicki sat in the front row of his class and copied his every word frantically while the other students tossed notes back and forth or tried to shield their bloodshot eyes from the painful florescent beams above.

In little ways Dr. Marley tried to help the misguided girl. Once, after a grueling test doomed to befuddle the most thoroughly prepared students, Vicki appeared at his office. At the time, Dr. Marley was on the phone closing a real estate deal on a new apartment. Unfortunately the girl had memorized his office hours and stood in the hallway with disapproving and accusing eyes as he spoke into the telephone. Dr. Marley kept talking, ignoring her gaze.

Putting one freckled hand over the receiver, Dr. Marley raised his head and said, "Please take a seat."

Vicki entered the room and primly sat on the edge of the chair.

"Yes?" Dr. Marley calmly asked, folding his arms before him after laying the receiver upon the hook.

Eagerly, her words tripping over her tongue, Vicki launched into a breathless review of the last test. " Is the Krebs' cycle interrupted at the point of carbon-monoxide combustion?" she asked excitedly, flipping the pages of her test until she came to page 8.

Startled, Dr. Harley was unable to respond. "I beg your pardon?" he said. Heavens, she didn't really expect him to know the answer, did she? Good grief, no one cared. In fact, he had taken that very section directly from an obscure, outdated textbook of his. It was his best trick. No student had ever been able to answer that question! It was his way of putting the graduating students in their proper places.

"Hmmm," he said. "Now what was the purpose of this visit?" That might throw the girl off the track.

OVERZEALOUS STUDENT

"Here," Vicki exclaimed. "On this question here, you placed a red mark, but as near as I can tell, the analysis I have presented is accurate. I looked all afternoon in the library but couldn't find the answer to this section on internal combustion anywhere. Why does the Kreb's cycle stop here?"

Dr. Marley stared blankly at the flushed face of his student with reserve. Well, he thought, perhaps flattery will work. Few women could resist a compliment.

"You know, my dear, you did extremely well on that last test! In fact, wasn't your score a 95," he praised. Then he sat back, relaxed. Surely she would giggle and lower her eyes. Perhaps he could sneak downstairs into the lounge and have a cup of coffee. He was still hoping to leave a little early since the Dean was on vacation.

Much to his bewilderment, Vicki leaned forward, placing her graded test on his desk. "Yes, I do have an A," she admitted, "but I still don't understand why you marked this section." Dr. Marley reached for the test. Then, turning the pages back to the front, he put an X through the 95 and changed it to a 100.

"My mistake," he admitted.

Puzzled, Vicki looked at the test. Still staring at the page before her, her eyebrows knit in bewilderment, she said, half to herself, "But it wasn't the grade that bothered me. I just didn't understand this." She looked at her professor with wide-eyed innocence and some confusion.

Those trusting, open wide eyes demanded a response. Firmly this time, Dr. Marley stood to his full height, pushing away from the chair.

"Ms. Kessler, you really must excuse me. I have an appointment and am already delayed. There is a complete description of the Krebs cycle in our library. Have the librarian check out a copy of Internal Combustion in Pharmacological Entities: Volume 27."

"Oh, thank you, Sir." Vicki said. How thrilling! He was treating her like an equal.

"I'll do so this very afternoon," she said.

MEMORIES OF A YOUNG PHARMACIST

When she left his office, Dr. Marley felt a twinge of guilt with relief. Well, he rationalized, it couldn't kill her to do a little extra library study. Next year he'd leave that question off his test. Hmm. He wondered now if anyone knew the answer to her question.

A good man at heart, and still concerned about the student's illness, Dr. Marley later tried to make it up to Vicki.

On the last day of class, he took a few moments to speak with her. Really, she was a nice child, despite her incurable zealous curiosity. "You'll be fine," he said, "as long as you just don't try to apply everything you've learned here…"

"Life isn't quite like it is in here - on campus," he kindly explained. How could he put in into words? Once out of the university, she would be met with a general lack of intellectual curiosity even in some of her peers, as well as the inevitable limitations imposed by time and energy.

Blind to his advice, Vicki left the university just as she had entered it. No, not just as she had entered. Worse. This time she had a cause. As she marched down the aisle in her graduating gown and black cap, she knew she was armed with pharmaceutical knowledge and apothecary wisdom. At long last, she was out of school and on the road to a career.

There was a world of suffering drugstore customers, a wealth of misguided prescribers awaiting the arrival of a clinical pharmacist. And tend them she would! She had memorized the Kreb's cycle, mastered the structural differences among the many benzodiazepines and phenothiazines, and could recite in a flash all the names of every tetracycline capsule marketed, bursting with knowledge and skill, this little lady pharmacist eagerly awaited her opportunity.

Oh, world of pill-users and abusers, she hummed happily to herself, here I come! Head held high, she proudly reached for her diploma along with the other pharmacy graduates that hot June day.

2

Patient Counseling - Very Patient!

Shortly after graduation Vicki began working at Nick's Drugstore in a cozy, rural town in Idaho. Vicki was nearly beside herself with joy. I've arrived! she repeated under her breath, pinching her cheek occasionally to see if she was dreaming. A diploma, a pharmacist's license, a real white jacket, and now this – a job!

During her first week on the job in the small, community drugstore, Vicki found herself faced with a real-life opportunity to counsel a patient. She was typing the label for a called-in refill when a tall, curly-haired male in his late 40's strolled up to the counter, his calloused hands casually tucked into his faded blue jeans.

"Where's yer Trojans?" he bluntly asked Michael, the 16-year old delivery boy.

Without pausing as he unpacked the United parcel drug shipment, Michael glanced briefly at the man and with a short jerk of his head he said, "She's the druggist."

Blinking in surprise, the man turned to look at Vicki. "You're in charge?" he asked, a slow smile forming at the corners of his mouth.

When the slender, blue-eyed girl nodded, he leaned both hands casually across the counter, laying his chin on it as his roving eyes appraised her petite figure.

"Well, don't that beat all!" he finally laughed. "Honey, I need some Trojans. Quit hiding back there and help me find 'em. I don't see 'em nowheres."

"Oh, well, Sir, state law requires the storage of contraceptive devices behind the counter," Vicki primly explained.

Then with a reassuring tone of voice, she added, "That's why you couldn't find them on the shelves."

She pulled open the white metal drawer before her and politely inquired, "How many Sir?"

"Ain't you going to ask me what size first?" the man asked, broadly winking at Michael.

Gulping, Vicki looked down at her feet and said in a small voice, "The manufacturer indicates that one size fits all."

"Hell, I'm not just anybody, pretty lady!" the man roared in laughter, "gimme a dozen."

As she handed them over the counter to the man, Vicki courteously said, "Michael will ring them up for you."

"Hey, ain't you goin' to tell me how to use 'em," the man asked in mock disappointment, grinning at Vicki. Then, jerking his thumb to the sign above the prescription counter, he read aloud, "We provide free counseling on the proper use of all prescriptions and supplies purchased here."

"Oh!" Vicki gasped, a hot red flush splotching her skin. She looked about frantically for Nick, her boss to come to her rescue. They hadn't told her about <u>this</u> in pharmacy school. Michael started to laugh.

I won't let this man get the best of me, Vicki thought. I am a professional person now, she reminded herself. Quickly pulling herself up to her full height of 5'1", Vicki faced the customer "man to man."

Chin held high, she pursed her lips together and, as though reproving a bad child, icily said, "If you don't know how to use them, you have no business purchasing them Good day!"

And with that she hid behind the shelves of prescription items, hoping that she had achieved a dignified exit, acutely aware of the man's eyes on her retreating figure. Concealed behind the shelves of drugs, Vicki smoothed the crinkles on her new white jacket, as the sound of the man's laughter slowly faded away.

3

Burying the Hatchet

Vicki was warned not to approach the physician. Warned not just once, but twice. With rose-colored glasses on, she completely ignored the warnings, convinced that she herself could judge this man better than his own partner in practice and the town druggist who had done business with him for fifteen years.

This physician was Dr. Growl. He was recognized in the community for his two most outstanding qualities: an explosive temper and excellence in his practice of medicine.

Seated in the Medical Director's office, Vicki explained her strategy to Dr. Stone, the 64-year old Medical Director and to Nick, the 48-year old druggist who had employed her to do chart reviews and drug audits in this nursing home.

"When Dr. Growl sees the quality of my work he will be really impressed!" she patiently explained to Dr. Stone and Nick. Carefully and earnestly she explained herself to these two men, who seemed to know so little about human relationships.

"You know, Vicki, Dr. Growl's temper is reputed to be so violent that even some of the experienced nurses out here avoid him," Nick cautioned.

Nodding her head Vicki listened, but let her thoughts fly freely. The reports were probably gross exaggerations, she surmised. In a small town gossips often made a mountain out of a molehill.

"Really Nick, there's nothing to worry about," Vicki said. "I've studied this man."

And so she had. She watched him when he made nursing home rounds, as she sat in safe anonymity behind the medical charts.

Dr. Growl was a short man- about 5'6" -almost Napoleonic in stature and stride, making his rounds briskly, head down as though rushing against a wind. His dark black hair was combed back and his blue eyes were clear and unblinking - the unfailing, immaculate, professional man in his white coat and starched shirt and tie.

Observing this dark-haired handsome man of medicine make rounds, Vicki more than once felt a haunting, fleeting sense of recognition. There was something about his dark, narrow 1940's moustache.

Suddenly one day when he entered the building it came to her. He looked just like Clark Gable! Both men were dark, blue-eyed, and adorned with thin, black moustache. Realizing who he resembled, Vicki felt safe. Clark Gable! The smooth-talking, romantic, eternal soldier of fortune and lover of women. So this was Dr. Growl's alter-ego.

Her silent, distant study of Dr. Growl went beyond the superficialities of public appearances. She sought to understand the man as a physician. Like a bloodhound, she examined all the available evidence.

His monthly notes were dry, factual statements.

Dr. Growl's elderly patients had an average of 4 drugs, compared to the overall national average of 6.4. His low drug use suggested careful, continuous monitoring of his aged patients. A perfectionist.

Month after month this lady pharmacist evaluated his drug prescribing, secretly hoping to "catch" him on something. How else could she introduce herself to him? With any luck at all, Vicki thought, I will find a really interesting drug-related point to bring to his attention.

Finally, in her third year of consulting, her perseverance paid off. She discovered a drug-related problem hinted at in the nurses' notes for for one of Dr. Growl's elderly patients. Aha, Vicki thought. This is it. Dr. Growl hasn't made his monthly rounds yet, so there is time to summarize my findings and contact him before his visit, she realized.

The professionally typed drug consultation in hand, she proudly shared it with Dr. Stone, the Medical Director and Nick, her boss.

Dr. Stone carefully read the cover letter and report. "It's medically sound." he said, closing the pages. Then he cautioned, "Now, you know, don't you Vicki not to expect anything but fireworks?"

Nick echoed the Medical Director's warning, then added, "Fine. Go ahead and send it. Just don't get upset when he starts throwing things and turns red."

With a sudden chuckle Nick added, "Yeah. That line about the Federal Government funding pharmacists to do drug reviews ought to make his blood boil!"

Cautious old-timers! Vicki thought as she sealed the manila envelope carrying the drug review. Really. Men had no imagination or powers of observation. The envelope was mailed to Dr. Growl's office on Monday.

Friday morning, Dr. Growl strode into the nursing home, immaculately attired in a form-fitting white jacket, with a stethoscope tucked into his lower right-hand pocket. He wore a brown and blue-striped tweed tie, which picked up the color of his vivid blue eyes perfectly.

Accompanied by the charge nurse who would make rounds with him, he briskly sat into a chair at the nurses' station. Silently he reached for one of his patient's charts, Vicki continued to work, hurt that he hadn't acknowledged her. Had he even read the review?

Suddenly she heard a deep masculine voice announce, "I got a letter the other day from the Federal Government."

With delight Vicki turned to face the handsome physician, who so resembled a movie idol. "What did you think of it, Doctor?" she expectantly inquired, leaning forward in her chair toward him. With both elbows resting upon her knees she cradled her chin in her hands.

Staring ahead Dr. Growl threw his pen against the counter where it hit with enough force to make Vicki jump back. His blue eyes blazed in blind fury and a splotchy red flush crept up from his collar to his cheeks. He spat his words out in an ugly manner.

"It's a violation of the doctor-patient relationship," he snarled. "Further more it's a complete waste of time and money. You stay out of my affairs and mind your own damned business! I've had it up to here with the Federal Government and you interfering agents!"

In growing horror the girl listened. A sick wave of nausea and anxiety swept over her. His hostile, furious words hit her again and again as she listened, in paralytic bewilderment and humiliation. While the young charge nurse behind them watched, an old arthritic ache complained.

Then Dr. Growl finished speaking as suddenly as he had begun. In the stark silence that followed the two warnings from Dr. Stone and Nick echoed again in the girl's mind.

Ignoring the rising bile in her throat Vicki lifted her chin and struggled for composure. With what little dignity she could muster, she spoke. "I'm sorry, Sir, to have offended you. Perhaps these reviews aren't of any benefit to you but the other physicians appreciate them."

Then refusing to admit complete defeat, she went on with the suicidal pride that had been with the Christian soldiers facing the lions in the ring.

"Well, how far should we go with this? I don't get paid any better when I contact the doctors with suggestions for patient care. I do it because I believe in it. If I mail another review to you, what will you do to me?"

He blinked his eyes, somehow taken aback. The silence now had softened and Vicki could hear the nurse behind her quietly breathing. Dr. Growl looked at the thin, pale young woman next to him. Her face was drained of color and her hands were clenched into fists. Good heavens, he thought, she looks like she's going to be sick. Maybe I was a little too emphatic.

Rising from his chair, while he reached for his stethoscope, Dr. Growl answered, "If you're right, I'll change my orders. If you're wrong, I'll call your boss and have your head and your job!"

When he had departed from the building, the 22 year old nurse who had witnessed their encounter advised, "Next time meet them on their own level." As she returned the metal charts to the rack the nurse went on to say, "Dr. Growl is very good with his cancer patients and even comes out at night to care for them when they are dying. He's a dedicated physician. I think he's huggable."

Huggable? Vicki echoed silently. Not to me. In all of my years of nursing home consulting I have never hugged a doctor, nor do I know anyone else who has.

Like a dog that has taken a bad, undeserved beating Vicki too turned mean and surly. When Dr. Growl entered the nursing homes, she avoided his gaze. If he stood near her to reach for a chart, she rose and grandly left the area. So it went for six months.

Then in May, during a routine review, she identified a significant and expensive drug-related problem on one of Dr. Growl's charts. His 64-year old patient was taking 30 ml of KCl daily in the absence of diuretics or steroids. If he changes the drug order, it will save his patient $30.00 a month, Vicki calculated. Then she caught herself. "Nope," Vicki told herself firmly. "Once burned, twice learned." She closed the chart and placed it heavily back upon the rack.

The following week she saw the same elderly patient approach the nurses' station with trembling, shaking hands asking for her Winston cigarettes. With a sense of shame Vicki looked away as the nurse lit the cigarette.

That harmless old lady takes two tablespoons of a salty, bitter liquid every day, Vicki realized guiltily.

With trepidation Vicki summarized her findings from the chart review and mailed the report to Dr. Growl's office. This time she knew what she was doing. The review went into the mail on Friday. The weekend passed. Then two more weeks. Still no response.

On the third week, Tuesday morning, Vicki went upstairs to her office in the drugstore. A note on her desk from the charge nurse said "Dr. Growl has made his monthly rounds."

On her desk sat a long white envelope. Opening it, she found her review with Dr. Growl's orders to discontinue the KCl. The physician had initialed it, and added the following hand-written salute: Touche!

Perhaps he wasn't huggable. But he was human and a healer.

She buried the hatchet.

4

Behind Closed Doors

Who said that group meetings must be all work and no play? Few people know what goes on behind closed doors when men of medicine work with today's young women.

On the last Thursday of each month, Vicki was released from her duties behind the counter of Nick's Drugstore to attend the monthly committee meeting in the town's largest nursing home. Although she was only twenty-three, Vicki had been entrusted with the handling of the nursing home account.

Nick, the drugstore's owner, liked the girl's positive attitude and hard work. Besides he enjoyed watching her walk about his store, reaching her slender arms upwards to place the prescription bottles back on the shelves. Despite her prim manner and the high turtleneck sweaters she wore, Vicki had an aura of good health and untapped sensuality. All in all, Nick found her to be an unusual resource for his business.

The nursing home Vicki consulted to, was being totally renovated.

The 50-year old Director of Nurses, was given a brand new office with orange-red curtains to match her long, painted fingernails. Vicki admired the changes and knew that it was just a matter of time before the patients' rooms were redone as well.

The rush of customers into the drugstore toward the noon hour had more than once kept Vicki from arriving on time to the monthly meeting. Apparently today was to be no exception.

"I'll be late again," Vicki nervously muttered, glancing at her watch as she hurried down the nursing home corridor to the conference room. The mahogany door was closed. Oh no. The meeting had already started.

"Well, better late than never," Vicki told herself as she turned the brass door handle to enter the room. She hated these late arrivals. Everyone stared at her when she walked in, making her feel more self-conscious than usual.

Timidly she stepped into the room which was already filled with the professional staff. Much to her surprise there was a visitor at the meeting. It was Lilly. Her nails were painted in the best of women's fashions. She sat firmly upright in her chair in the corner of the room, legs crossed and a pen professionally held in hand, ready to take notes.

But it was Lilly's incredible summer blouse that stopped Vicki's entrance into the room. Swallowing hard, Vicki stood momentarily transfixed in the doorway, her hand still gripping the doorknob for security. She was caught off guard.

A hot, uncomfortable flush traveled across Vicki's adolescent chest up to the collar of her jacket, rising over the edge of her turtleneck sweater. Try as she might, she simply couldn't quite lift her eyes from Lilly's blouse to meet the gaze of the others in the room. She was held there for only a few seconds, but in that spellbound state, time stood still.

Lilly's white blouse was dangerously low cut. A scalloped collar dipped seductively in a V-shaped line to reveal a hint of Lilly's sumptuous cleavage. Tiny pearl buttons dressed the front, precariously tugging the blouse about the woman's body. Those shiny pearl buttons mirrored the fluorescent lights above, winking and twinkling as they teased each man in that hot, stuffy conference room.

Yet it wasn't this flimsy, delicate blouse that anchored one's eyes. In frank, unabashed availability smiled two full, ripe breasts proudly smiling. When Lilly turned in the chair her starched blouse crinkled, creating ripples of sound that conveyed the woman's hot, repressed desire. In concert with the most subtle movements of Lilly's shoulders, her breasts also swelled and undulated like a buoy upon a wavy lake.

In the muggy, airless room a faint, seductive hint of perfume floated above the table over the metal charts, beckoning the male faces back toward that blouse. With the ancient wisdom of Eve in the garden of Eden, this woman sat in complete silence. Yet her invitation was more articulate and more inviting than mere words could ever have conveyed.

Vicki's hypnotic spell was suddenly broken by the Medical Director's authoritative voice. Looking up from his bowl of soup, Dr. Stone raised his grey bushy eyebrows commanding Vicki's attention.

"Late again, huh, kiddo? Pull up a chair and sit down. Soup's getting cold."

Vicki gracefully closed the door behind her and slipped into the empty chair.

Then she turned toward the facility's new administrator, apologetically stammering, "I'm terribly, terribly sorry. But I just couldn't get away on time. The relief man didn't come in until noon. Then one of our best customers came in to return a battery just as I was starting to leave the store. I told him that I was already behind time, but he..."

"In other words you were unavoidably detained?" the young man smoothly interrupted her.

"Oh, well yes, I guess that's what I'm trying to say," Vicki demurred, lowering her eyes in embarrassment to the bowl of soup before her.

The room was silent again, except for the occasional sounds of spoons clattering against china soup bowls and coffee poured into cups. Vicki set about eating her chicken noodle soup, careful not to let a single drop slip unnoticed down her chin or onto her pharmacy jacket.

Cautiously, Vicki raised her eyes from the bowl of hot soup and carefully peered out at the men in the room. All of them were nicely eating lunch. Not a single one was taking sneak peeks at the Medical Records supervisor.

As the meeting progressed, Vicki's embarrassment faded and in it's place stirred curiosity and a kind of jealousy. I could never pull off an outfit like that! she thought. Besides my husband, John, would never let me out of the house in that blouse. Guess God gave me more brains than body, she sighed in disappointment. By 12:30 both Dr. Stone and Dr. Grin, the 40-year old family practice physician, began to pull metal charts from the neighboring tray onto the conference table. Coffee cups and bowls were moved to the side. The sound of spoons and dishes were replaced with voices discussing patient care.

"Mrs. Jones still on skilled nursing care? I can see from her progress notes that the decubitus ulcer has healed and that she is eating in the dining room now," Dr. Stone remarked. He lifted his eyes from the chart to peer above his horn-rimmed glasses to glance at Lolita.

"Oh, well, let's see now," Lolita said, leaning toward him, lightly placing her manicured fingernails upon the shoulder of his tweed jacket. "Doctor, I do believe you've got a point! Yes, indeed, she should be moved to Intermediate Care…Hmmm. Guess that's one chart I just overlooked."

Dr. Stone initialed "ICF" on the medical records review sheet and closed the chart, taking another one from the stack of metal charts before him. As he opened the next chart, he glanced at the list of medications on the doctor's order sheet.

"Hey, Vicki, here's one for you to field," he said. "What's this thioridazine stuff good for? Does it cause shakes like Haldol did in my last patient?"

Vicki leaned forward, eager to fulfill her role as a clinical pharmacist. At last, a question she could field. Taking a deep breath, she began, "Well, actually, Sir, the entire class of phenothiazines are not at all alike. The carbon on the central ring plays a significant role in determining the eventual effect of the drug upon the dopaminergic-cholinergic system. Thioridazine is highly effective in the elderly and mentally retarded patients as a moderately sedating psychotherapeutic agent. But yes, you are quite right, Doctor, in ascertaining that it has a potential for depleting dopamine stores in susceptible patients." Finished, Vicki sat back in her chair, her hands primly folded upon her lap, a pleased smile touching her lips.

Dr. Stone lifted his head to gaze at the young woman. Firmly and decisively he lay his pen down upon the mahogany table. Then he carefully closed the chart and folded his hands before him as he raised his gray eyebrows.

'Thank you. Brilliant! Madame Curie couldn't have done better. But I didn't understand a single word."

"Now, let's try again, my dear Victoria. Will this drug cause pseudo parkinsonism in my patient or not? And why is he taking it? I'm not even sure he needs it."

Thus finished, Dr. Stone nodded his head curtly and picked up the metal chart again.

"Oh," Vicki gasped, her composure shaken by the physician's confrontation. "Well, gosh! I'll sure find out why he's taking the drug when I complete my drug history. And, oh, yes, it can cause pseudoparkinsonism, but is less likely to than Haldol."

"Thank you, my dear," Dr. Stone remarked, his blue eyes twinkling with humor as he picked up his pen again. A lovely girl, he thought. A mind like a scientist and the lithe, eager little figure of a skater. If only she could learn to be more concise.

As usual, the meeting adjourned at 1:00 when both physicians departed for their offices. Vicki went out to the central nurses' station and began her afternoon's review of the medication sheets.

Briskly settling into a neighboring chair, Lilly remarked conversationally, "Heavens! I'm already behind schedule. I was supposed to fly out to our California facility this afternoon, but I simply must finish the audit here before survey next week. But then that puts me quite behind my work in our Oregon and California homes. It's getting to be quite a challenge keeping up with all of the homes facilities," Lilly sighed as she brushed a lock of hair out of her forehead.

"What an exciting life you lead. Your job is quite unusual for a woman, too," Vicki quietly responded in secret envy.

"Yes, I just adore my work. I meet the most interesting people and have complete independence," Lilly smartly declared flicking a speck of dust off her dark red nails as she tossed her head back.

The two women sat side by side quietly working. Once again Vicki felt a wave of self-reproach as she compared her uneventful life and uneventful dress with the woman next to her.

Then as if speaking to herself, Lilly added, "But you know, I think I could give it all up if I could just get married again like you."

Vicki lifted her head to look again at the sophistocated, well-groomed woman. Suddenly she dropped her eyes to the linoleum floor, her mind ringing with a similar admission made by another woman in another age.

It was Elizabeth Marbury, an American theatrical agent, born in 1856 who caught the moment with her remark, "A caress is better than a career."

5

The Doctor and The Fly

"Some of our more confused residents are known to wander into open rooms," Maude explained as she closed the mahogany door to the nursing home's conference room. Despite the oppressive heat of the desert summer, the committee members would be forced to endure the muggy atmosphere until the luncheon meeting was adjourned.

Vicki gave an inaudible groan. Well, just can't be helped I guess, she decided. Then she began to eat lunch, tugging restlessly at her high-necked cotton collar. Lunch usually proceeded the nursing home's committee meetings. The fare was trim.

"I do hope you enjoy our little snack today," Maude brightly announced. "We're all on diets," she explained daintily reaching for a tiny sandwich. It wasn't clear to any of the other committee members what exactly Maude hoped to accomplish on her diets, since she had a pleasing figure at her age. But when the administrator dieted so did the rest of the professional staff.

As the meeting progressed a kind of light-headed weakness began to overtake Vicki. She too had a battle with weight, but hers was on the far end of the spectrum. She barely tipped the scales at 115 pounds, giving her the appearance of perpetual adolescence. The only thing big about Vicki were her large, expressive eyes.

After this meeting is over, I'm going to pick up a real lunch at

McDonald's, Vicki promised herself. I simply won't make it through the rest of the afternoon shift back at the drugstore on this thin fare.

Fatigue and hunger pangs began to set in, although it was barely 12:30. Vicki stifled a rude, revealing yawn as she shifted uncomfortably in her chair.

The committee members pushed their plates to the side as the business was brought forward for discussion. A series of complaints were raised, the most pressing being the nature of the pharmacists' responses to emergency calls from the nursing home. In the suffocating heat of the airless room, the angry debate between the nursing staff and pharmacy ensued.

Lolita, the Director of Nurses, led the attack on pharmacy, "We've simply got to have drugs when we need them!" she insisted, her heavily made-up face contorted in frustration and barely concealed rage.

Just the other night one of the drugstore's pharmacists had been summoned for "call duty." The charge nurse had awoken the slumbering man at midnight and demanded immediate delivery of a drug.

"Mr. Jones is constipated. We have no Ex-Lax in any of the unit dose drawers," she complained.

More tired than tactful, the sleepy druggist had muttered, "Sorry, lady, that ain't no emergency," and had placed the receiver back on the hook.

As it turned out, the patient had eventually received a glass of prune juice, with good results, but the damage had been done. By the time Vicki arrived the battle lines had been drawn. Before Vicki could rise to the defense of her fellow pharmacist, Dr. Jones interceded with a practical, non-partisan suggestion.

"Why not build a crash kit or an emergency board?" he asked, hurriedly signing his patient's chart before returning to the office. "At the hospital they have some kind of kit. I could check into it and let you know." he offered.

"Well, we already have an emergency kit with over 50 items," Vicki helplessly explained, "and replacements are being made daily."

With the peevish look of a spoilt child who has been ignored, Lolita insisted, "Yes but the kit is never adequate to meet our special needs. For example, some times we need Castor oil, or maybe NuGauze, or the patients might want cigarettes from their accounts, or, or , well, all sorts of things." She paused to collect her wits, unable to offer an adequate defense for her cause. Then, inspired, she turned to face the Medical Director.

"If the Doctor orders something, we've simply got to have it! Don't you agree, Dr. Stone?" she sweetly asked, drawing the Medical Director into the argument, as she lightly traced her fingertips along his knee.

Lolita had enlisted his help just in time!

The meeting was rapidly drawing to a close. Dr. Stone had exactly five minutes to resolve the debate. All eyes turned to this man. Maude anxiously twisted her hands in her lap, upset by any conflict between the professional staff. Lolita eagerly looked at Dr. Stone, hoping that her appeal had won the war for nursing. Karen, the medical records assistant, held her pencil tightly in hand, ready to record his every word.

Vicki sat across from the sober, unsmiling physician, intently listening to his concluding remarks. Her slender hands were folded upon her lap. Beads of perspiration formed across her forehead from the tension of the debate and the humid, muggy atmosphere in the room.

Silence fell as the Medical Director pushed his coffee cup aside, placing his broad surgeon's hands upon the table. He cleared his throat. The soft chirp of a sparrow on the bush outside broke the silence. No one spoke.

Just as he began to speak, a fly entered the open window, droning around the physician's crown of silver hair. Why the indignity of it! There was not a living soul in that room with the nerve of the fly, threatening to interrupt the Medical Director as he made his concluding comments.

Suddenly the light lunch and heat began to affect Vicki's nerves. As she stared at the figure of authority before her, swatting at that little fly, a frightening desire to giggle overtook her. Suddenly she snorted. Quickly, she raised a napkin to her lips to smother the outrageous laughter that threatened to erupt in the hot, overcrowded conference room.

Dr. Stone lifted his eyes to glare at Vicki, his stern, forbidding face cold and expressionless as usual. Maude shot Vicki a quick, angry look to silence her.

"Please excuse me, Sir," Vicki choked, pretending that she had sneezed. She bit her lip forcefully and pressed her nails into the palms of her hands until they ached, silently praying, "Oh, God, please, please don't let me laugh."

As she dropped her eyes to the floor she recalled the wise adage, "There are few men who would not rather be hated than laughed at." Dr. Stone continued to speak with great clarity and authority. Without pausing in his comments, Dr. Stone lifted his strong former basketball-player's hands to his head and tried to swat that fly. His first two attempts to combat the attack of the little fly had failed. This time the fly returned to circle his grey head with a vengeance!

Reaching his broad hand upward in a smooth and decisive fashion, Dr. Stone grasped the insect in mid-air, his hand pausing for a second to crush the impudent offender. Without so much as a blink of the eye or a twitch of his grey eyebrows, he opened his large hand and dropped the fly upon the carpeted floor, still speaking with great calm and dignity.

As he concluded his final remarks, he lay both broad hands back upon the conference table. Much to her embarrassment, Vicki abruptly realized that she had no idea what he had just said.

The whole moment, the man's entire address on pharmacy services, had been completely eclipsed by his ability to catch the fly!

In sudden panic, Vicki realized she had missed the entire message. What would she tell Nick? What was it that the Medical Director had said? She cast her eyes about the room, nervously searching the faces of the other committee members in the hope of finding the answer. Too late. They were all moving away from the table. She anxiously twisted her hair in one hand.

And then, thankfully, reason returned to the girl. She remembered that the meeting minutes were recorded. She could find out tomorrow.

Vicki returned the next day to the nursing home and pulled the black notebook onto the conference table, turning the pages until she finally found a summary of the committee minutes. Dr. Stone's bold, masculine voice of authority rang out in strength on the typed page before her:

"A joint meeting with the pharmacy committee required a considerable portion of time. Discussion -regarding 'Emergency pharmacy cases' attempted to delinete from the pharmacy standpoint, the criteria of emergency.

Having given this review some thought, I feel that pharmacy is in no position to determine the emergent nature of requests for medication. Rather this is a problem for the attending physician and/or nursing supervisor, either of whom should be empowered to request emergency service.

While it is admittedly an imposition on the pharmacy on rare occasions, theirs is a position of service to the Care Center, and should be accomplished as efficiently and timely as possible."

Thus concluded the Medical Director.

And not a single word about the naughty fly either, Vicki giggled!

6

The Perfect Gentleman

"Hey, let's have Vicki make rounds with us this morning!"

Vicki felt a quick rush of pleasure and pride when Dr. Stone nodded in assent. They were treating her like one of the guys. Maybe Dr. Stone was beginning to take her work seriously after all.

Tugging self-consciously at her clinging skirt, Vicki followed the two men down the linoleum hallway. Ken held the metal charts in his hands, along with a notebook of recorded concerns to bring to Dr. Stone's attention. As they walked along, Ken called over his shoulder, "Yeah. You'll really like this new patient, Vicki. He's in restraints from slugging two night aides. Guy must weigh 200 pounds. And cuss....! You're the first woman we could get to go with us..."

Oh, so that's why they invited me! Vicki thought hotly. It wasn't a professional compliment at all. They just needed a fall-guy for their practical joke. Now what do I do? Simply follow the fellows down the hall like a guinea pig? Turn around and admit that I don't like swearing either? Many stroke patients in the nursing homes lost their inhibitions and some were known to utter the most offensive, abusive things.

An old man was restrained in his wheelchair. His yellowish-white hair was combed back in a kind of style more fashionable in the late 1950's than in 1980. Signs of tardive dyskinesia were already evident, even at a distance, by the man's slow repetitive tongue protrusions and the prancing motions of his lower limbs. His face was rough and leathery, his nose large and red.

As they arrived at the man's side, Dr. Stone reached into his suit jacket for the stethoscope.

In a sudden, inspired move - destined to reverse the practical joke, Vicki stepped before the new admission. Squatting low onto her haunches, she placed one hand upon the man's shoulder, smiling directly into his blue eyes.

"Hi. My name's Vicki," she began in a low voice. "These fellows think you're going to embarrass me by cussing a blue streak, but I believe that you'll act like a perfect gentleman."

And then she coaxed, "You just show them how to treat a lady."

There was silence. The old man slowly extended his gnarled hand toward Vicki, his cloudy blue eyes vague and somewhat unseeing. He didn't speak, but a smile touched his mouth as he placed one hand on hers. Vicki stroked it softly for a moment, adding, "You'll be happy here once you get used to it."

Then she rose and turned to Ken, lightly saying, "You could learn something from these patients...." And with that, she quickly made her escape down the hall, back to the safety of her medication sheets and charts.

Vicki never did hear this patient swear in her presence. Coincidence? Maybe. However, she was convinced that even this 78-year old man, impaired by his years of drinking and a stroke still wanted to live up to the expectations of a young woman.

Maybe he too knew that "Kindness is a language which the blind can see and the deaf can hear."

7

His Kingdom for a Car Ride

This Tuesday's staffing proceeded no differently than any of the others had.

The professional staff had reviewed the care plans and short-term goals for the four residents and started to disband. Just as Vicki gathered her purse and notebook together, she saw a nose appear at the archway of the door.

Slowly following the nose was the aged face of Charlie, one of the nursing home's most mysterious residents. His frozen, expressionless face and hooked, beak-like nose were eerie. And today, on the eve of Halloween, it was downright spooky. The old man looked into the room, where the staff were still seated.

His abrupt appearance and departure startled the group. In comic relief the attending physician, Dr. Ward, chuckled and burst out, "He's the perfect Boogie man! I'm going to take my kids down here tonight and warn them to be good or HE'LL get 'em."

Jackie, the middle-aged Director of Nurses, frowned in silent reproof at Dr. Ward's remark. Yet she had to admit that Charlie's slow, shuffled walk and gaunt face did resemble the terrifying Boogie man depicted in so many children's stories.

No one knew much about old Charlie. He never spoke to anyone and never smiled. In face, his mouth was turned down in a permanent disapproving scowl. There was not even a twinkle in his eyes to suggest a spark of life or humor.

Odd as it seemed, Charlie was a wealthy man. At the age of 89, this man with a 60-year history of psychiatric and institutional care of "Chronic, undifferentiated Schizophrenia," had a bank account of $200,000.00! His only work record was from a 3-month tour of duty in the army in 1917. All of Charlie's income came from his service-connected disability, resulting in a steady accumulation of wealth over the past 60 years.

Now, at the vulnerable, venerable age of 89, Charlie was in his final, twilight years. His one true pleasure in life was car rides.

Cara, a 20-year old grandniece, was Charlie's sole surviving relative. Although low on cash, Cara was rich in time and compassion. Each week little Cara arrived at the nursing home dressed in her snug blue jeans and velcro-closing sneakers ready to chauffeur solitary, scowling Charlie. The girl's dilapidated 1964 rambler with the dented front door was Charlie's ticket to unmitigated freedom and sinful pleasure.

A slight smile threatened to touch the corners of his mouth when he sat by Cara, breezing along at the incredible speed of 30 miles per hour. Around town this unlikely couple would sail, up to the city's rim and down through the empty shopping districts on Sunday. Out and about they would fly in delicious, forbidden pleasure.

Then one day the fun was over. Observing the sorry state of Cara's car, the facility staff reluctantly decided it wasn't safe for Charlie to ride in it any longer. And so the car rides were stopped.

Silent, severe Charlie sat in his solitary world in the nursing home, without interruption.

Moved in compassion for her patient, Jackie sought to release a small amount of Charlie's fortune so that Cara could purchase another car. After all, little Cara would inherit all of Charlie's $200,000.00 upon his death. And at his age, this was an imminent possibility.

So the proceedings began. Each month Jackie wrote to the main Veteran's office in Michigan, seeking a release of some of her patient's funds. Each month she completed and filed a 4-page form. Legal counsel was obtained on Charlie's behalf. For 2 years, monthly letters were sent for release of funds.

Finally in February 1984, Vicki left the nursing home, but the drama continued. Before she left the facility she stopped at Jackie's office, asking, "Did you ever get a release of funds for Charlie?"

In exasperation and frustration Jackie looked up, opening her hands in apology. "No," she finally admitted, "but I haven't given up...."

On her way down the hall Vicki saw old Charlie seated in the lounge, his vacant eyes fixed upon the television set, still waiting for his car rides.

Poor little rich man.

8

The Kiss

"That's it!" Vicki exclaimed, lifting her eyes up from her paperback book to look at her husband John. "I should have been born a man I wish I were one," she added ruefully, chewing on her fingernails.

Without looking up from his newspaper John dryly asked, "Wouldn't that put a certain strain on our marriage?"

With a laugh Vicki dropped the book onto her lap. "What I mean is that I do a man's job. As a pharmacist, I work with men and try to work equally hard. But I'm not a man. Things would be so much easier if I were one."

"I think Freud had a name for that kind of envy," John rejoined. Then he continued, "Grass is always greener, Vicki."

"Still, I think life is easier for men," Vicki stubbornly insisted. As if to prove it, she lifted her book to show her husband the book's cover - <u>Dress for Success</u>. "Right here it says if a woman's going to be a success, she's got to dress like men, act like them and never let them know that she's a woman. At least I think that's the overall message," she concluded.

"Well, then if you read the Hollywood exposes you'll find out that some women undress for success, Vicki," John said. "Why don't you just try being yourself?"

Later when Vicki had finished reading <u>How to Win Through</u>

THE KISS

<u>Intimidation, Women at the Top and Dress for Success</u>, she had to admit that the different formulas weren't without drawbacks. Sometimes when she was dressed all correctly in the recommended gray tailored suit, seeing the overcast gray skies of late winter, as she reviewed the sad medical histories of some of her nursing home patients, Vicki felt the cold press of still greyness seep into her soul.

"You know Vicki, you used to be a lot more fun before you took yourself so seriously," the medication nurse remarked one morning as she reached into her cart for a bottle of Colace. "Remember those crazy hats you used to put on? The patients love 'em."

In a sudden, uninhibited move, Vicki bought a new hat!

It was a beauty. Made of soft, white, woven straw, it curved to fit her head perfectly. Around the edge it was trimmed with black velvet ribbon and a black feather waved from the top. Perfect, Vicki decided.

"How do you like it, John?" Vicki asked that night, slowly turning in a circle so that he could admire it from all angles.

"Terrific! You look just like Robin Hood," he chuckled.

Undaunted, Vicki proudly wore her new hat to the next pharmaceutical services committee meeting. Walking into the building, she was stopped by an older wheelchair-bound woman. "Ohhh," the woman sighed, "Ladies used to wear hats all the time. You look sooo stylish honey."

Secretly pleased Vicki thanked her and entered the conference room like a queen, taking her usual seat next to the Director of Nurses. The two women made small talk as they waited for the arrival of the second physician, Dr. Beldon. Opening the door, he entered with his usual aplomb and big smile. Then he stopped, stared at Vicki and said, "Getting awful formal aren't we."

With a whoop of laughter, he pulled the hat right off Vicki's head and held it over the table. The curved, straw hat cupped in his hands, he asked, "May I have my salad in this today?"

With a sniff, Vicki thrust her chin forward and said defensively, She added, "My son said I looked beautiful in it."

The older physician looked at the hat, back to Vicki's face, and said, as he placed the foolish hat back upon her head, "Well, and so do I!" Then much to Vicki's shock, he sat down in the chair next to her and kissed her cheek.

The room broke up in laughter as Vicki flushed uncomfortably. The 58-year old Administrator, tightened up. "At our last survey, our cook Ruby served hot cinnamon rolls to the team of Federal Surveyors. One of the men kissed Ruby right on the cheek. It was most unprofessional!" the woman coldly remarked, glaring with disapproval at Dr. Beldon. Crisply she added, " I sent a letter of objection to his superiors in Washington!"

Uh, oh, Vicki realized. She's jealous. Dr. Beldon was known for his bedside charm and striking good looks. Well-built, dignified and humorous, this physician had more than once been the secret heart-throb of many a romantic young nurse and lonely female patient.

"Well, thank you, Sir," Vicki murmured. "When I write my memoirs I'll put this incident in them."

Dr. Parsons, a silver-haired neurologist, looked up briefly from his charts to growl, " How to handle senile old men in the nursing homes?"

Any man who finds me attractive can't possibly be senile, Vicki thought, carefully adjusting her hat.

After the meeting Vicki went to the nurses' station to begin her monthly reviews. Dr. Beldon finished making his monthly rounds to his nursing home patients, pausing to write new orders. When he finished, he spoke to Vicki, asking, "Was there a special occasion you were dressing up for?"

"Oh, well. No. It sort of cheers me up," Vicki explained in confusion, the black feather on her hat waving and bobbing as she spoke.

"You know," the man finally said. "It can be a lonely life for a woman who tries to be a man in a man's profession and a man's world. I see this all of the time with the women physicians."

Embarrassed at his insight, Vicki looked away, and then added, "No matter what, I guess I never will be one of the guys."

Dr. Beldon slowly shook his head. Turning slightly to the side, he went on to say, "When you fill us in on these drug reactions, you talk like a man. In fact, it seems to me that you think like one. But you'll always feel and look like a woman." Then pausing to clear his throat he said, raising his eyebrows slightly, "However, it your case that's an occassion for good cheer."

"Oh!" Vicki startled, a small flush of delight filling her cheeks.

With a short nod, Dr. Beldon headed down the hall and out of the building. With the black feather bobbing Vicki dropped her head and returned to her work. Maybe it wasn't such a bad hat afterall.

9

Drugstore Robbery

Vicki returned from her summer's vacation refreshed and invigorated. Camping in the high, crisp cool Colorado mountains had brought a fresh color to her usually pale skin.

"Hey, ready to get back to work?" Marc called out in greeting as Vicki sailed into Nick's Drugstore.

"Sure, always," she replied. "Anything exciting happen while I was gone?" she asked, absently sorting through the stack of mail lying on the prescription counter.

Marc paused to look up at her. "Matter of fact, you did miss the excitement. The store was robbed - armed robbery. And the very weekend I was on call, too."

"Robbed?" Vicki repeated, looking up. "Anyone hurt?"

"No," Marc replied. "We were tipped off in time. It was an inside job." Turning his back to Vicki so he wouldn't have to see her face he lightly added, "Michael set it up."

"Michael!" Vicki gasped. "Not our Michael?"

"Yeah," Marc replied, moving away from her side. Darned females. Always on the verge of tears. Made him nervous.

Dropping the mail from her hands, Vicki slowly walked to the back of the store and up the stairs to her office. Michael? A criminal?

She sat down heavily into her chair, her bouyant, vacation-mood replaced by sober reflection. Michael's serious, vulnerable face rose before her. Of all the high school kids who had worked at Nick's Drugs, Michael had always been her favorite.

From a poor family, Michael had been forced to work long hours down at the store, after school and on week ends to help pay the family's bills. Yet, even with the long hours he put in he had graduated with honors just a few weeks ago.

Michael had been protective of Vicki, never letting her carry the shipping cartons of drugs to the back of the store. Whenever Vicki had night duty, Michael had remained at the door with her until the heavy glass doors were securely locked. He had even seen Vicki safely to her car in the darkened parking lot. Once in awhile she caught him looking at her. The woman in Vicki cherished his youthful naive admiration for her.

Shortly before Vicki's vacation the store employees had given Michael a big party for graduation. He had been accepted into the state university's pharmacy program. Along with his many gifts was a new PDR from Vicki. "I sure will use this! Just need to be able to understand it," Michael exclaimed in pleasure as he impulsively reached over to hug Vicki.

Now with a police record what chance was there for him to follow through on his dreams? Vicki wondered. Who would ever give him a job in any drugstore? Had life fated this boy to forever living on the wrong side of the tracks, with no avenue of escape?

After work Vicki casually approached Marc, asking "What really happened? I mean about Michael?"

"Grab a cup of coffee," he said and gently added, "It kind of upset all of us. Nick's taking it the hardest. He won't even talk about it."

Marc sipped his coffee and settled into the aluminum folding chair in the back of the store. Vicki sat next to him, ready to hear the story.

"Well it was on Saturday night," Marc began. "I was carrying the beeper. At about 2:00 am the police called and woke me up. They told me that the pharmacy was going to be robbed by an employee. They had been tipped off by an inside informant."

"Someone knew?" Vicki asked in surprise. "Who?"

"Police won't reveal the identify of the informant. But Michael owes quite a lot to that person." Marc answered.

"What do you mean," Vicki interrupted. "What's the informant have to do with it all?"

"Hold on. I'm getting to that part," Marc went on "The police were tipped off earlier and have been watching the store - a couple of plain clothesmen have been on the job."

"We've been watched?" Vicki asked uncomfortably.

Marc nodded. "Anyway that Saturday night one of their men, lying in a van in the parking lot, saw a car drive up. They saw Michael get out, unlock the store at midnight and walk in."

"But the alarm," Vicki interrupted, puzzled. "Why didn't the alarm go off with his entrance."

Acknowledging her remark by a short nod he explained, "Michael didn't have a key to turn off the alarm box, but he knew the system inside out. He figured out a way to jump over the electronic beams or reset them using mirrors around the store to redirect their paths."

Vicki shook her head in disbelief, seeing young Michael's figure in the blackened empty store on a Saturday night.

"They arrested Michael a few minutes later as he was coming out the back door.

"Now here's where Michael got lucky. Since the police were tipped off in time, Michael was charged only with breaking and entering. He's not a minor anymore you know. An hour or so later, the guys who had engineered the robbery arrived with shotguns and cleaned out the scheduled drugs. Police caught 'em a block from the store. They were charged with armed robbery - a felony and a mandatory jail sentence."

A cold chill touched Vicki's spine as she recalled other nights when she herself had opened up the dark, deserted store late at night to fill emergency drug orders. And to think that she herself could have walked into a situation like that.

"But how did Michael get involved? Why? I mean, he had his whole life, his college career before him?" Vicki asked.

"Breene, the kid that set it up has held up other drugstores in the area. Smart kid, in his late 20's. Anyway this Breene met Michael at a party and found out he worked for Nick. So Breene started dating Michael's sister. She was the one that finally talked Michael into it."

"He dated Michael's sister just so he could make a contact into the store?" she repeated, a slow cold awareness dawning.

"Evil isn't it?" Marc agreed. "Breene promised Michael $10,000.00 to get a duplicate key, open the store and walk away. Hell, that's about it," Marc abruptly concluded, slapping his palms down upon his knees.

Eyebrows knit in worry, Vicki asked, "What's going to happen to Michael now? I mean, no job, a police record, no college?"

Look Vicki, he's not your responsibility," Marc reminded her. "I know you liked the kid. We all did, but he's a big boy now."

But the serious, vulnerable face of the blonde boy-man wouldn't leave Vicki. The next day, with her heart in her hands she approached Nick, against her better judgment and Marc's advice.

Standing at his side she said, "Nick, can I talk to you?"

"Shoot," he muttered, adjusting the Brunswig screen to read the entries.

"It's about Michael," she started hesitantly.

"Vicki, he got just what he deserved."

"But, Nick, he's still so young," Vicki said. "He's like my younger brother."

"Jesus Christ almighty!" Nick shouted. "What the hell do you expect me to do Vicki?" he asked as he started thumping her shoulder with a pointed finger. "Give the kid another key and invite him into the store so's he can hit it up one more time?"

Vicki swallowed, dropping her eyes to the floor silently crying.

His jaw fiercely set, Nick wheeled away and stormed to the back of the store. Women, he muttered. Enough to drive a man to drink.

The next morning, before the store's doors were unlocked, Nick walked in with Michael. He had just taken the boy out to breakfast. "Hey, crew come over here," he commanded the store employees.

MEMORIES OF A YOUNG PHARMACIST

"Kid's going to help me work on the house," he roughly told his employees. "Can't use him down here now, but I need a strong arm out at the place."

By the end of the summer, after 45 job applications, Michael was finally granted an interview, by the owner of a sugar beet factory. The police record had worked against him, making most employers shy away from an unnecessary risk.

Finally a job on the night shift - for minimum wage - appeared. The owner contacted Nick, who wrote the following letter of recommendation:

Michael Easton has been a loyal, hard-working employee of mine. He's courteous, intelligent, and eager to please.

For reasons not clear to me, and I'm afraid tragically unclear to the boy himself, he was involved in an attempted burglary of my store this summer.

He remains on parole. Over the summer he has worked for me, doing yardwork and construction. Again I found him to be an excellent worker and I highly recommend him. He's one of the finest teen-agers we've had in our store.

Michael got the job. In six months he was promoted. Within two years he found a job driving a UPS truck.

One day Vicki shyly approached Nick. "Nick," she began, "You know I've never told you how much I admire you for your work in pharmacy... I mean, that was terrific when you were the Pharmacist of the Year! And, wow, incredible when they gave you the Archambault award for your nursing home reforms."

"Um, get to the point kid," Nick said absently. "You looking for another raise?"

No," she continued. "You've received more honors than any other pharmacist I've ever met. But as long as I live I will always remember you as the man who gave Michael a second chance," she said as she reached a slender arm around his expansive waist to hug him.

"Urr," Nick muttered, pulling uncomfortably away. "Never could stand to see a female bawl. Go home Vicki, before I put you to work again."

10

Til Death Do Us Part

Once in awhile I realize I'm a human being and I want to stay with someone for longer than a night, or a week for 'forever' the way my grandmother used to put it.

Anonymous

The rising incidence of divorce among American couples is like a national epidemic. Doesn't anybody stay together any more? Upon Vicki's desk were gifts from her girlfriend - a stack of womens' magazines, thirteen in all. All of them address marital discord, techniques for preventing affairs, and sex secrets for married woman wanting more romance, sex or fidelity from their husbands.

The titles of the articles in these popular women's magazines reveal our insecurity:

"What makes sex better? Love last? 12,000 couples share the secrets of intimacy."

"Formula for a Happy Marriage." - "Stop Fighting and start loving again."

"How we saved our marriage" - "The five sex secrets men are afraid to share."

Can we uncover the mystery of love in of a magazine?

But Vicki witnessed the fulfillment of this pledge in the nursing

MEMORIES OF A YOUNG PHARMACIST

homes. This, then, is the love story of Senna and Bill Marks, who made this pledge in 1937 and lived it.

The nurses station was in the center of the brightly lit, new building.

By slowly turning in a circle Vicki could see all of the four hallways which led away from this center into the patient's rooms.

Each Thursday morning at exactly 10:10, an immaculately attired man would slowly pass by Vicki, pushing an older woman in a hand-crafted wheelchair. Sometimes he would speak to the woman or smile, after bending down to hear something she had said.

Down the hall and about the building he and the older patient would stroll, a kind of hypnotic rhythm in their slow, unhurried travel.

At first Vicki thought the man was a devoted son, pushing his aged mother. Their age difference was marked. Her gray, curly hair was like that on a doll. She looked paralyzed - unable to move, beyond the smallest turn of her head.

One Thursday when he slowly went by Vicki commented upon the beauty of the hand-made quilt around the woman's shoulders. He paused to speak with Vicki, politely and formally thanking her.

"I see you hear every week," Vicki said and went on to praise him, "You're a good friend."

Leaning over to smile upon the silent woman restrained in the wheelchair, he gently corrected Vicki by tenderly saying, "You've been the best of friends to me, too."

With a slight smile and a nod, he then continued down the hall, slowly pushing his wife.

When there was a lull in the activities Vicki asked the charge nurse about this couple. For the past 2 years this 64 year old woman had been in the nursing home. She was almost totally crippled by severe arthritis, unable to dress herself comfortably. Unable to walk. The blue eye which seemed so lifeless and expressionless was a glass eye. Her health problems were so severe that her husband had been unable to care for her any longer at home. Finally, he was forced into admitting his total care wife into the nursing home.

He himself was a wealthy man, a retired realtor whose investments and sales were so monumental that he could afford to pay, in cash, for his wife's monthly nursing home bill which totalled $1,500.00.

Mr. Marks was a handsome man, in spite of his years. By some he would have been considered still a "good catch." Yet this man chose to spend his days pushing the wheelchair of his crippled wife. He seemed tender and gentle with her, often helping the nurses with her care, brushing her soft curly hair and applying her make up.

As time went on, he and Vicki spoke occasionally. Sometimes he would simply walk by, on his way out of the building and with a smile, show her the white envelope containing his monthly drug bill. That bill alone came to $150.00 a month.

Once in awhile he'd stop and comment on the weather or tease Vicki about working too hard. One day Vicki stopped him and asked him about his life with Senna.

"Well you just stick with it. Senna has a terrible temper, but once she's mad, she's done. When I'm mad, I pout. We just never got angry at the same time. You just stick with it. I don't know what I'd do without her."

Then with his usual polite smile and nod, he went on out of the building.

'Through sickness and through health, for better or for worse, 'til death do us part.'

11

Can We Be Honest? - Selling Clinical Services

"There's a new administrator out at Happy's Home for the Aged," Nick casually told his pharmacists. "I think I'll just check things out, before I meet the guy. The secret in business is to be able to out think your opponent."

Later that week, Nick went out to check the emergency drug supply, determined to work the nursing home grapevine to his advantage. Norma usually helped him, that is to say, she stood in the drug room with him, swapping stories between sips of her coffee. Good old Norma. A farm girl at heart - with a soul as big and broad as her ample bosom and manly shoulders. The Hoyer lift had been designed with Norma in mind. But where the Hoyer lift was known to be faulty and recalcitrant, old Norma and her back would never give out.

"Norma, doll, you're the best doggoned nurse around," Nick said, leaning over the counter at the main nurses' station. "Any chance I can get you to open up that emergency kit for me? Got some replacements for you too," he added, holding up the paper sack as proof of his sincerity and good will.

"Well, I was just about ready to call the doctor back for orders on our new admission," she grumbled. "Oh, all right, all right," she muttered heavily pulling herself out of the chair.

She reached for her mug of steaming coffee before deserting her post at the main nurses' station and led Nick around the corner to the small closet which contained the emergency kit. Pulling the keys out of her uniform pocket, she reminded Nick, "It's the one with red on it."

With a deep breath and a manly shrug of his shoulders Nick stepped forward to face the music. Darned E. Board! There were now 50 items listed! Well, here we go. He began the itemized check of alphabetized items:

2-Adrenalin 1:1000

Yes, they were all there. And expiration date still current.

1-Calcium Gluconate injection. O.K.
5-Digoxin 0.125 mg tablets Nope, only 3.

"Norma, where is the missing dig?" he called over his shoulder.

"Oh, yeah, guess I forgot to let you guys know. He used two of them pills today. Mr. Roard spit his out this morning and Mabey had her dose increased, so we just doubled up on her."

The aides pushed the carts of dinner trays down the hall, rattling by noisely as Nick continued to check the board. Finally he concluded the job.

"Thanks Norma. You can lock her up now," he said.

As she turned the key in the lock he asked as nonchalantly as possible, "What's this I hear about a new head boss taking over? Know anything about the man?"

"Someone's been waiting in the wings now for a few months," Norma admitted, slowly turning back toward the nurses' station. She took a sip of her coffee, then, fortified, she continued, "He's a young one, they say. Plenty of education- smooth talker, the whole bit. They call him 'The Stud,'" she cackled, her large bosom heaving in appreciation.

"The Stud?" Nick asked in astonishment, stopping in his tracks to stare at her in bewilderment.

"Look it up in Webster's, Nick," Norma laughed. "Doubt if you'll find it in the PDR. Gotta call the Doc now 'for it's too late," she said, turning into the nurses' station.

Thus dismissed with no more information, Nick puzzled over the nickname.

Stud? A womanizer? No, they'd never advertise that. Must be a man's man Nick decided. A straight shooter would be a relief. No beating around the bushes, quibbling over nickels and dimes. Could put all the cards on the table.

Tucking his hands into his pockets as he headed toward his car Nick felt a sudden lift. Old Nick's not so dumb after all. Got all the dope I need on the new guy.

The "Stud" arrived before Nick's repeat check on the E. Board. Two days after the new Administrator's arrival, 3 of the floor nurses quit. He fired the activity director and rumor had it that he was actually interviewing physicians for the Medical Director's post. As they say "A new broom sweeps clean."

Within four days of his arrival, the pharmacy services were called forward for an accounting. However, Nick remained confident. Didn't he have more awards than any other druggist in town? Hadn't his clinical pharmacist made in-roads with these hard-core independent docs? Not a single check mark against them on survey for the past 10 years, either.

Nick dressed up for the meeting with the new administrator. He was kept fully waiting, outside the main office. Finally after an interval of 40 minutes he was ushered into the administrator's office.

"Please. Take a seat," Mr. Young generously offered, his open palm pointing to the plush new chair across from his desk.

Just as Nick started to praise the new painting hanging behind the man, the administrator abruptly spoke.

"I'm short on time. Let's get right down to brass tacs," this thin, balding young man insisted.

CAN WE BE HONEST? - SELLING CLINICAL SERVICES

"Well, now, that suits me just..." Nick began comfortably.

"Your pharmacy services." Mr. Young interrupted. "Costing us too much. Got to cut back somewhere." he firmly concluded placing both hands on his desk.

"Well, we certainly want to remain competitive, but after 12 years of business with your center, we feel we've got the best there is to offer." Nick said.

Calmly "The Stud" pulled a 2-page form out of his desk drawer. "Here, he commanded, handing it across the desk to Nick. "Fill this out. We want a complete and itemized accounting of your pharmacists' time in our facility. And see to it that your people get physicals and T.B. tests. Need those reports next week."

With a slow sense of numb shock, Nick looked up at him. Was he serious?

"We put in about 35 hours a month," he explained, "but we've never been asked to explain our role. Why - the docs know how helpful these clinical services are! Just last week, for example, Vicki sent a review to Dr. Homes that prevented some serious side effects. And when we added the cost savings from this work, why we've saved the patients over $350.00 in drug bills last month alone! The way that gal works so hard she's going to put me right out of business."

Abruptly "The Stud" looked at his watch. "Hmm, well, excellent," he responded, "I'd like that form by next week," he repeated. "In fact, none of the home's consultants will be paid until these forms are filed. Got to go now," he finished, rising from his chair.

Stunned, Nick clamored to his feet, blankly looking at the form in front of him.

"Thank you Sir for your time." Nick said. As he left the office in a daze, he muttered, so this was "The Stud."

When he returned to the drugstore he called Vicki, Marc and Rob together. "Fellahs," he said in a hearty voice, "we get some free medical care with this new administrator. We all gotta have physical exams. But the Medical Director will provide them .

Rob looked up with distaste, raised his eyebrows and muttered,"You tell that joker that I'll show him mine, if he'll show me his." And with that he wheeled around the corner to answer the phone.

Despite the resistance by his professional staff, Nick finally cowed his pharmacists into compliance. Either they complete the form and secure physicals or else!

Duly submitted, all forms and physicals were filed on Monday. On Thursday, Nick received a letter from "The Stud" announcing the termination of all pharmaceutical services. Service closure date was in 3 months.

"Sorry, honey," Nick said to Vicki, "but I still gotta send you out there to do the last of the reviews. Stiff upper lip and all that. You never know, the contract might swing back this way next year."

As instructed, all services were provided until the final day. Vicki carefully went over her check list, marking off the items.

Gathering up her purse and notebook, she prepared to leave the building.

On her way out "The Stud" stopped her asking, "May I have a minute of your time?"

Vicki entered his office and sat down. Hands on his knees, the thin, balding man leaned forward and asked, "Can we be honest?"

Try it, you might like it, Vicki thought with humor. But she simply nodded and said, "Certainly."

"Well," the administrator explained, "your boss insisted that you guys put in 35 hours a month. Now I see you each week, but those figures are outrageous! Why it can't take more than an hour to sign those sheets. Who does Nick think he is kidding?"

"Mr. Young, with all due respect, Sir," Vicki said firmly, "Nick isn't kidding you at all. We take our jobs seriously."

"I wasn't trying to insult you," he smoothly continued. "Your work is highly regarded. "But honestly, 35 hours?"

"Honestly," Vicki said quietly. "You may never see a clinical service like this again.

Still puzzled, "The Stud" looked at Vicki. "Why does it take the druggist so long to look at the chart?" he finally asked.

"Well," Vicki patiently explained, "He has to see to it that the drugs are given in the right doses and correspond with those charted on the medication sheets. And then he or she must read the progress notes."

"The progress notes!?" Mr. Young interrupted."That's ridiculous. Why is the druggist reading the progress notes?"

Helplessly Vicki shrugged her shoulders. "To find out if there are any drug-related problems."

"Hm" the man sighed. "'Why can't you just sign the charts like I asked? I can see we're getting nowhere," he peevishly concluded, standing with his hand outstreched.

"Our best wishes with your new providers." Vicki said, shaking the offered hand.

Still puzzled "The Stud" stared as Vicki walked down the hall. She seems honest,he thought, and convincing. Something didn't add up.

As she left, Vicki thought, we still aren't reaching the powers that be.

When Vicki left consulting, she wrote the following story: called, "The Doctor who refused to grow old."

12

The Doctor Who Refused to Grow Old

Dr. Ward Stone, a man 40 years my senior, touched my life only briefly; however, his integrity and sweep of spirit captured my unguarded heart.

In a small farming town, in the spring of 1978, I met this 65-year old physician, whose care of the frail elderly revealed to me "all that rings true, all that commands reverence, and all that makes for right." (Phil. 4:8)

In addition to his full-time family practice, Dr. Stone also served as the Medical Director to the nursing home where I had recently been employed. My job in the local facility was to notify the Medical Director of problems identified through review of the patients' charts. Fresh out of college, I embraced my work with all of the zeal and idealism my 30 years of living afforded. Yet, all that I truly knew of either nursing homes or the practice of medicine, came from college lectures and textbooks. With the naivete of youth, I plunged headlong into a confrontation with Dr. Stone- the hospital's former Chief of Staff.

Around 10:00 that spring morning, I looked up from the desk to see an imposing man quickly approach the nurses' station, accompanied by the charge nurse.

So this was Dr. Stone - an angular and forceful-looking man with thick gray hair. His energetic stride and slim figure defied his 65 years.

He paused momentarily to glance in my direction, as he reached for a chart.

"Now or never," I told myself, heart racing furiously. Tale-tell signs of anxiety were apparent.

"Doctor...."

From his towering height of 6'4", Dr. Stone turned his fierce, penetrating eyes toward me, unblinking and expressionless. He sized me up mercilessly, much as the eagle stares at the terrified field mouse scurrying below.

"Now that you've opened your big mouth," he thundered, "what have you got to say for yourself!"

Even now I don't recall exactly what it was that I said. I know that I stammered and stuttered and finally managed to complete my thoughts. When I had finished, Dr. Stone withdrew his intimidating, relentless gaze from mine. He abruptly turned his back to me, acknowledging my input with a curt, "I'll think about it."

I was frankly grateful that the "showdown" was over. I felt a flush of relief sweep over me.

In the five years following this initial encounter with Dr. Stone, I never did feel completely at ease in the presence of this exacting, formidable man.

Eventually I learned that no one escaped Dr. Stone's hawklike scrutiny. In his own relentless fashion, he kept all of us on our toes. Anyone failing to meet his exacting standards of excellence could expect to be brought up short and in clear, unequivocal terms.

I recall the hurt outburst of a nurse who had been sharply criticized by Dr. Stone: "He's arrogant, obstinate and rude!" she muttered, furiously slamming her charts upon the formica counter. After a few minutes, I overheard her admit with a reluctant sigh, "However, I suppose that's part of the charm of the man."

Dr. Stone freely stormed into other people's affairs if he felt corrective action was indicated. At one committee meeting in the nursing home, I watched Dr. Stone begin his assault upon the 35-year old physician who sat across from him.

Raising his gray eyebrows slightly, while continuing to sign the papers in front of him, Dr. Stone declared, "Didn't I see you leave the office the other night at 5:00? In 40 years of practice, I never left that early! People can't always be sick from 9 to 5, son."

Not content with embarrassing a fellow colleague in public, Dr. Stone went on to remind the nursing home administrator of his duties as well. "I discovered a tray of cold food leaving your kitchen the other night when I was out here." Dr. Stone sharply accused the man. "Most of these people spend the day looking forward to their meals. No matter how old you get, you still want a hot supper," he abruptly reprimanded.

Soon afterwards a system for checking the temperature of food trays leaving the kitchen was established.

Stories of the blunt and forthright Dr. Stone rippled through the small town, provoking an inevitable smile in the listener.

It was a startling relief to meet a man who didn't mince words. Here at last was a man whose actions and beliefs could not be contained by social niceities or public opinion.

Seated at the nurses' station early one morning, I overheard a prim nurse in her late 30's consult with Dr. Stone about her recent abdominal distress. After detailing her physical complaints at length, she asked Dr. Stone for his opinion.

"Well, are you pregnant?" he began, as he pulled his patient's chart from the rack.

"Dr. Stone!" she gasped, coquettishly lowering her eyelashes. With a suppressed giggle, she added, "I'm not even married. How could I possibly be pregnant?"

"Only one way I've ever heard of," he dryly responded.

For better or for worse, Dr. Stone had a pronounced effect upon others. One of his nursing home patients, a 74-year old woman confided, "My doctor terrified me at first. He's very blunt you know, that little rascal! But I believe he's about the best doctor in town."

THE DOCTOR WHO REFUSED TO GROW OLD

His intimidating presence was noticed by his patients in the community as well. One young computer programmer admitted with a grin, "If Dr. Stone can't cure you, he'll scare you into getting well!"

Despite his blunt and relentless criticism of nursing home caregivers, Dr. Stone showed a warmth and patience with his elderly patients. In his care of these people, there stood another sort of man. As he spoke to a confused old man restrained in a wheelchair, Dr. Stone's relaxed, open face assumed a kind of beauty.

"It takes a certain kind of courage for a doctor just to walk into these places," Dr. Stone once admitted in a rare moment of personal reflection.

Whatever else the plight of the nursing home elderly stirred in this man remained unexpressed. He continued to visit his patients regularly three mornings each week. The nurses told me that he also went out to the nursing home at all hours of the night for emergency calls.

Dr. Stone's devotion to the care of the frail elderly awoke something in me. At the age of 53, Dr. Stone had worked in the battlefields of Viet Nam with Project Hope. At that time he was the only physician available to treat civilian war casualties in a province of 250,000. Almost twenty years later he remained the same, outspoken, unswerving moral man. Only now his dedication to medicine thrust him onto the silent battlefied in the nursing home. I often imagined that he was daring old age or ill health to catch up with him.

My feelings for this dedicated doctor were captured in a passage from <u>Years of the Locust</u>. The author seemed to be describing me as well, when she wrote about the fierce devotion a young woman felt for her powerful, outspoken grandfather "Old Dade," when she wrote that "her very disposition made her be close to him, as young and old can occasionally become, ignoring all differences in age and sex, seeing only a oneness of spirit."

I found sketches of aged nursing home patients, called <u>Images of Age</u>. The artist, Michael Jacques, had sketched these portraits while visiting his own Grandfather in the nursing home. I carefully dressed my present in bright wrapping paper decorated with dainty sprigs of red flowers, mistletoe and holly. Then I had my gift delivered to Dr. Stone's private residence.

After Christmas break, I saw Dr. Stone in the nursing homes again. In a characteristic fashion, he strode by me as I sat quietly working at the nurse' station. Briskly he turned around and shortly stated, "By the way, thank you. I read your book."

And then lifting his chin higher, he proudly insisted, "I could have written a better one!"

"Well," I wryly reminded myself, He's not the sort of man to sit down a write a flowery thank-you note."

The holiday seasons passed and imperceptibly the weeks and months slipped by. When Dr. Stone announced his retirement from private practice, I wondered if he would leave the nursing home as well. Little did I realize that I was soon to leave.

In the spring of 1982 my employer lost the contract to serve the nursing home where I had worked for five years. In short, I was dismissed. No farewell parties. No good-byes. Nothing. The closing date of service drew near.

I felt a heaviness of spirit descend upon me, despite my intention to view the lost contract as a simple business reversal. I continued to submit my reports to Dr. Stone, who seemed unaware that our association was drawing to a close.

The night before my final day in the nursing home, I felt a turbulence of emotions. Fatigue, disappointment, and hurt pride and having been "fired," clouded my thoughts and strained my heart. Memories from the past five years surfaced unbidden. I remembered the 93-year old man who missed his invalid wife so much that he "kidnapped" her from the nursing home. I relived the scene of a woman stricken with Huntington's chorea who one day miraculously walked down the hall, upheld by two assistants. I could see again the look on Dr. Stone's face as he bent over to listen to a wheelchair-bound patient speak. Other images and memories tugged at my emotions. That night I tossed about in restless sleep on a tear-stained pillow.

The morning of the last day arrived. With fresh resolve to hold my thoughts and feelings in check, I went out to the nursing home for the last time. I was working at the nurse's station when Dr. Stone arrived.

"Quitting are you?" he barked, giving me a sidelong glance as he entered the nurses' station where I sat.

"Not exactly," I quietly replied.

He sat alone at the nurses' station in front of the rows of hanging metal charts. Dr. Stone began pulling his patients' charts from the rack and stared thoughtfully at one he had opened. With his eyes still intently fixed upon the chart below, he slowly offered, "Well, I'll miss you."

Then he lifted his gaze to look at me with a smile. "That's something, you know," he gently volunteered, "when you're missed." His face held the relaxed, open expression I had seen reserved for his elderly patients.

My throat tightened suddenly in fresh ache and disappointment. Tears blurred my sight. I blindly reached out for his waiting hand and pressed my cheek against his. For the briefest of seconds I felt the warm touch of the man I had come to love, drawing comfort in his strong, near presence.

Then Dr. Stone briskly rose, turned down the hall, and returned to his battle with old age and ill health.

I saw Dr. Stone once again one sunny Fall afternoon while I was walking with my five-year old daughter to the public library. He was stepping out of the church when our paths crossed. My heart quickened in familiar recognition.

As he walked away, I told my daughter excitedly, "That's the doctor who takes care of the Grandmas and Grandpas in the nursing home!"

She looked up and bluntly asked, "Does he know that he's old too?"

I glanced over my shoulder, watching him stride swiftly away. Then I turned to her with a smile, answering, "No, honey. I think that man refuses to grow old."